STRETCHING EXERCISES FOR SENIORS OVER 60

10 Minutes Daily Exercises For Men And Women To Relieve Back Pain, Improve Balance And Posture And Reduce Risk of Injury

Christina J. Whitley

Copyright 2023, Christina J. Whitley

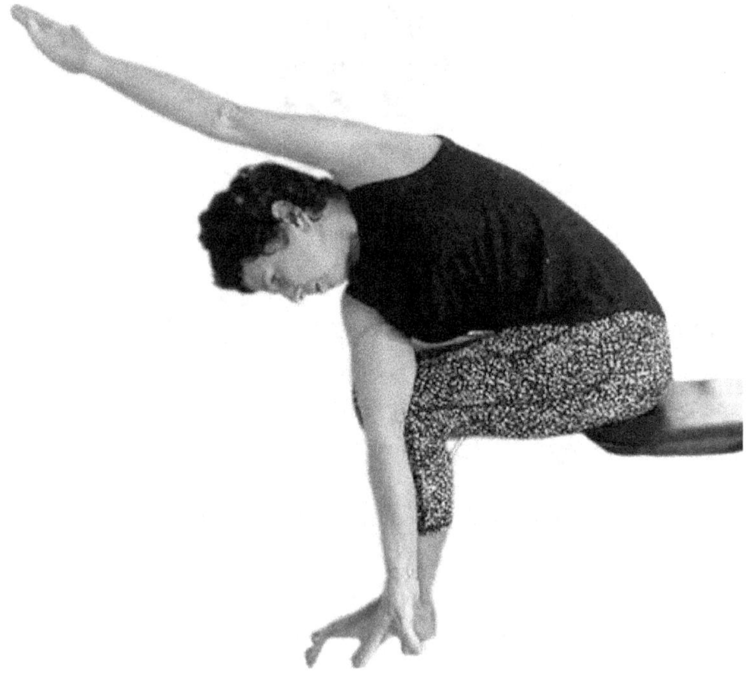

Table of contents

INTRODUCTION

There lived an extraordinary woman named Eleanor in the center of a peaceful senior community. She had just turned seventy years old, and with every year that went by, she started to notice physical changes. Her once-steady balance had begun to falter, her strength was failing, and her flexibility looked like a far-off memory. Eleanor felt that the secret to regaining her youthful vitality was in finding the appropriate stretching exercise program.

One bright morning, Eleanor made the decision to go out on a quest to address her worries. Her mission was to learn the techniques for recovering mobility, strength, flexibility, and balance. Searching for the ideal manual to help her return to the route of wellbeing, she perused countless books, articles, and internet resources.

After weeks of determined research, Eleanor discovered a thorough stretching exercise guide specifically designed for seniors. It seemed to hold the key to the renewal she'd been looking for. She took the guided home and, full of hope, decided to give it a shot.

Eleanor was exposed to a multitude of exercises and strategies by the guide, which she could attempt on her own. She accepted the task with a fierce determination, prepared to resurrect her strength, enhance her flexibility, restore her balance, and expand her mobility on her own.

Eleanor turned each page of the guide and discovered a myriad of exercises that targeted every area of her body She started her journey by stretching her tight muscles, slowly but surely regaining her flexibility. The tension in her shoulders and neck, which had become all too familiar, began to melt away.

With each exercise, her legs and core got stronger as she followed the guide's easy-to-follow instructions. She was astounded at the increased strength in her gait and the ease with which she could get out of a chair.

Her breath was taken away by more than simply the physical changes. Her life was made more peaceful by the guide, who taught her how to meditate and do deep breathing exercises. Once shattered by unrest, Eleanor's sleep deepened and became healing. Her once unsteady balance got better with each practice, increasing the comfort and security of her everyday life.

As they observed Eleanor's metamorphosis, her friends, family, and fellow seniors were astounded. She demonstrated firsthand how a suitable guidance for stretching exercises could lead to a plethora of advantages. Her friends were inspired by her adventure and ready to follow her example, while her husband John witnessed his wife blossom with life.

Eleanor's narrative provided a powerful reminder that being older shouldn't ever be a hindrance to wellbeing. With the correct stretching exercises manual, you may change your life, get back your flexibility and strength, and enjoy your golden years with health and vitality. She had found her own spring of youth and urged others to follow in her footsteps. Eleanor's narrative served as a timeless example of the amazing advantages of having the ideal guide, direction, and self-determination.

The journey of life is a remarkable and enduring adventure, filled with experiences, wisdom, and an ever-evolving sense of self. As we gracefully navigate our way through our golden years, one key factor remains undeniably essential: the well-being of our bodies and minds.

For seniors over 60, the benefits of regular stretching exercises are nothing short of transformative. These exercises hold the power to enhance not only physical flexibility but also mental clarity and emotional equilibrium. They enable us to rediscover our strength, regain our balance, and relish the freedom of movement that brings joy to our daily lives.

In this comprehensive guide, we will explore the art of stretching for seniors over 60. We will delve into the countless advantages that regular stretching can bestow upon you, from reducing muscle tension to enhancing posture, improving sleep quality, and promoting overall physical and mental well-being.

So, if you are eager to embark on a journey to unlock the secrets of aging gracefully, we invite you to join us on this exploration of stretching exercises tailored specifically for seniors. With dedication and guidance, you will unearth the fountain of youth that lies within the simple yet powerful act of stretching, setting a course for a life rich in vitality, balance, and the joy of well-earned wisdom.

CHAPTER 1

Why Stretching is Important for Seniors:

1. Improved Flexibility: Stretching helps maintain and enhance joint flexibility, making it easier to move and perform daily activities.

2. Reduced Risk of Injury: Regular stretching can prevent muscle and joint injuries, especially in older adults.

3. Enhanced Range of Motion: It allows for a wider range of motion, making it easier to reach, bend, and move comfortably.

4. Better Posture: Stretching can help correct posture problems commonly seen in seniors.

5. Pain Relief: It can alleviate chronic pain conditions, such as arthritis and back pain.

6. Balance and Stability: Stretching improves balance, reducing the risk of falls.

7. Stress Reduction: It promotes relaxation and reduces stress, benefiting mental health.

8. Increased Blood Circulation: Stretching can enhance blood flow, which is crucial for overall health.

9. Improved Sleep: Seniors often find that stretching can lead to better sleep quality.

10. Independence: Maintaining flexibility and mobility allows seniors to remain independent and active in their daily lives.

Safety Considerations For Stretching

1. Consultation: Always consult with a healthcare professional before starting a stretching routine, especially if you have underlying health conditions.

2. Warm-Up: Begin with a gentle warm-up to prepare your muscles and joints for stretching.

3. Proper Form: Maintain proper form during stretches to avoid straining or injuring muscles or joints.

4. Pain-Free Stretching: Stretch to the point of tension but never to the point of pain.

5. Breathing: Incorporate proper breathing techniques to support relaxation and prevent dizziness.

6. Gradual Progression: Start slowly and gradually increase the intensity and duration of your stretches.

7. Stay Hydrated: Drink water before and after stretching to prevent dehydration.

8. Safety Equipment: Use props or support like a chair or wall for balance if necessary.

9. Cool Down: Finish your stretching routine with a gentle cool-down to help your body recover.

10. Listen to Your Body: Pay attention to your body's signals; if something doesn't feel right, stop and seek guidance.

Basic Stretching Principles

1. Warm Up: Always start with a light warm-up, like gentle cardio or dynamic movements, to increase blood flow and prepare your muscles for stretching.

2. Proper Form: Maintain correct posture and alignment during stretches to avoid straining muscles or joints.

3. Gentle and Slow: Stretch slowly and gently; avoid sudden or jerky movements to prevent injury.

4. Breathe: Incorporate deep, controlled breathing to relax and enhance the effectiveness of your stretches.

5. Hold Stretches: Hold each stretch for at least 15-30 seconds to allow your muscles to relax and lengthen.

6. Progressive Overload: Gradually increase the intensity and duration of your stretches as your flexibility improves.

7. Balance Both Sides: Stretch both sides of the body equally to maintain balance and prevent muscle imbalances.

8. Focus on Major Muscle Groups: Concentrate on stretching major muscle groups to improve overall flexibility.

9. Stretching Routine: Develop a consistent stretching routine to make it a habit and see long-term benefits.

10. Listen to Your Body: Pay attention to your body's signals; if you feel pain or discomfort beyond gentle tension, ease off or modify the stretch.

CHAPTER 2

Neck and Shoulder Stretches

1. Neck Rolls:

- Sit or stand with your back straight.

- Slowly tilt your head to one side, bringing your ear toward your shoulder.

- Gently roll your head forward, then to the other side, and finally back to the starting position.

- Repeat this circular motion for 15-30 seconds in each direction.

2. Shoulder Rolls:

- Stand or sit with your arms relaxed at your sides.

- Roll your shoulders forward in a circular motion, lifting them up toward your ears, then rolling them back and down.

- Perform this movement for 15-30 seconds and then reverse the direction.

3. Gentle Neck Stretch:

   - Sit or stand with your back straight.

   - Tilt your head to one side, bringing your ear toward your shoulder.

   - Gently use your hand to apply slight pressure to increase the stretch.

   - Hold for 15-30 seconds on each side.

4. Shoulder Blade Squeeze:

   - Sit or stand with your arms at your sides.

   - Squeeze your shoulder blades together as if trying to touch them behind your back.

   - Hold for 15-30 seconds, then release. Repeat a few times.

5. Upper Trapezius Stretch:

   - Sit or stand with your back straight.

   - Reach one arm over your head and gently touch your opposite ear.

   - Gently tilt your head to the side, using the weight of your hand to increase the stretch.

   - Hold for 15-30 seconds on each side.

CHAPTER 3

Upper Body Stretches

1. Arm and Chest Stretch:

- Stand with your feet shoulder-width apart.

- Extend your arms straight behind your back, interlock your fingers, and gently lift your arms.

- Feel the stretch in your chest and shoulders.

- Hold for 15-30 seconds and release.

2. Back Stretch:

- Stand with your feet hip-width apart.

- Interlace your fingers in front of you, palms facing out.

- Round your upper back, pushing your arms away from your body.

- Feel the stretch across your upper back.

- Hold for 15-30 seconds.

3. Torso Twists:

- Sit on a chair with your feet flat on the ground.

- Cross your arms over your chest.

- Slowly twist your upper body to one side while keeping your lower body still.

- Hold for 15-30 seconds on each side.

4. Doorway Stretch (Pectoral Stretch):

- Stand in a doorway with your arms bent at a 90-degree angle and your forearms against the doorframe.

- Gently lean forward to feel the stretch in your chest and the front of your shoulders.

- Hold for 15-30 seconds.

5. Shoulder Blade Squeeze:

- Sit or stand with your arms relaxed at your sides.

- Squeeze your shoulder blades together as if trying to touch them behind your back.

- Hold for 15-30 seconds, then release. Repeat a few times.

CHAPTER 4

Lower Body Stretches

1. Leg Stretches:

- Sit on the floor with your legs extended straight in front of you.

- Reach forward and try to touch your toes or ankles.

- Hold the stretch for 15-30 seconds, feeling the stretch in your hamstrings and calf muscles.

2. Hip Flexor Stretch:

- Kneel on one knee, with the other foot in front, forming a 90-degree angle.

- Push your hips forward slightly while keeping your back straight.

- You should feel the stretch in the front of your hip.

- Hold for 15-30 seconds on each side.

3. Ankle and Calf Stretches:

- Stand facing a wall or a sturdy support, with your hands against it.

- Step one foot back, keeping it straight, and press your heel into the ground.

- You'll feel the stretch in your calf and Achilles tendon.

- Hold for 15-30 seconds on each leg.

4. Seated Leg Stretches:

- Sit on the floor with your legs extended straight.

- Bend one knee and place the sole of your foot against your inner thigh.

- Reach forward toward your toes on the extended leg.

- Hold for 15-30 seconds on each side.

5. Butterfly Stretch:

- Sit on the floor with your feet together and your knees bent outward.

- Hold your feet with your hands and gently press your knees toward the floor.

- Feel the stretch in your inner thighs and groin.

- Hold for 15-30 seconds.

CHAPTER 5

Balance and Stability Exercises

1. Standing on One Leg:

- Stand with your feet hip-width apart.

- Lift one foot off the ground and balance on the other.

- Hold for 15-30 seconds and switch to the other leg.

- You can make it more challenging by closing your eyes or raising your arms to the sides.

2. Heel-to-Toe Walk:

- Position one foot directly in front of the other, heel to toe.

- Take slow and deliberate steps, walking in a straight line.

- This exercise challenges your balance and coordination.

3. Chair Exercises for Balance:

- Stand behind a sturdy chair or use a countertop for support.

- Lift one leg slightly off the ground and balance on the other.

- Hold for 15-30 seconds and switch to the other leg.

- As your balance improves, try letting go of the chair for short periods.

4. Leg Swings:

- Stand next to a wall or a support.

- Swing one leg forward and backward while keeping the other foot on the ground.

- The swinging leg should not touch the ground during the exercise.

- Do this for 15-30 seconds on each leg.

5. Balance Board or Pillow Stand:

- Stand on a balance board or a soft pillow with one foot or both feet.

- Try to maintain your balance while keeping your core engaged.

- This exercise challenges your stability and strengthens your core and leg muscles.

CHAPTER 6

Seated Stretches

1. Seated Leg Stretch:

- Sit with your legs extended straight in front of you.

- Reach forward and try to touch your toes or ankles.

- Hold the stretch for 15-30 seconds, feeling the stretch in your hamstrings and calf muscles.

2. Seated Torso Twist:

- Sit with your legs extended in front of you.

- Cross one leg over the other, placing your foot flat on the floor.

- Gently twist your upper body in the direction of your crossed leg.

- Hold for 15-30 seconds on each side, feeling the stretch in your lower back and hips.

3. Seated Upper Body Stretch:

- Sit with your back straight.

- Reach both arms overhead, interlock your fingers, and turn your palms upward.

- Stretch upward and to one side, feeling the stretch along your side and arms.

- Hold for 15-30 seconds on each side.

4. Knee to Chest Stretch:

- Sit with your legs extended straight.

- Bend one knee and bring it toward your chest, hugging it with your arms.

- Hold for 15-30 seconds on each leg, feeling the stretch in your lower back and hips.

5. Seated Butterfly Stretch:

- Sit with your feet together and your knees bent outward.

- Hold your feet with your hands and gently press your knees toward the floor.

- Feel the stretch in your inner thighs and groin.

- Hold for 15-30 seconds.

CHAPTER 7

Full-Body Stretching

1. Standing Cat-Cow Stretch:

- Stand with your feet hip-width apart.

- Inhale, arch your back, and lift your head and chest (Cow position).

- Exhale, round your back, and tuck your chin (Cat position).

- Repeat this flowing motion for 30 seconds, moving between Cat and Cow stretches.

2. Forward Bend with Arm Circles:

- Stand with your feet hip-width apart.

- Reach your arms forward, bend at your waist, and let your upper body hang.

- Slowly circle your arms in one direction for 15 seconds, then reverse the direction for another 15 seconds.

3. Deep Hip Flexor Stretch:

- Kneel on one knee, with the other foot in front, forming a 90-degree angle.

- Gently push your hips forward while keeping your back straight.

- Hold for 30 seconds on each side to stretch the hip flexors.

4. Full-Body Stretch with Reach:

- Stand with your feet shoulder-width apart.

- Reach your arms overhead, interlocking your fingers and turning your palms upward.

- Stretch upward and then lean to one side, feeling the stretch along your side and arms.

- Hold for 15-30 seconds on each side.

5. Seated Butterfly Stretch:

- Sit on the floor with your feet together and your knees bent outward.

- Hold your feet with your hands and gently press your knees toward the floor.

- Feel the stretch in your inner thighs and groin.

- Hold for 30 seconds.

CHAPTER 8

Relaxation and Mindfulness: Breathing and Meditation Techniques

Relaxation and mindfulness techniques are valuable additions to any stretching routine, promoting not only physical but also mental well-being. By incorporating practices that center your mind and enhance relaxation, you can enjoy a holistic approach to your overall health. Here are some breathing and meditation techniques to consider:

1. Deep Breathing:

- Sit or lie down in a comfortable position.

- Inhale slowly through your nose for a count of 4.

- Hold your breath for a count of 4.

- Exhale slowly through your mouth for a count of 6.

- Repeat this deep breathing pattern for a few minutes to reduce stress and calm your mind.

2. Mindful Breathing:

- Pay close attention to your breath as you inhale and exhale.

- Notice the sensation of the air entering and leaving your nostrils or the rise and fall of your chest.

- If your mind wanders, gently bring your focus back to your breath.

- Practicing mindful breathing can improve your concentration and reduce anxiety.

3. Body Scan Meditation:

- Close your eyes and take a few deep breaths.

- Mentally scan your body from head to toe, focusing on each part and releasing tension.

- Begin with your forehead, then move down to your neck, shoulders, and so on.

- This technique promotes relaxation and self-awareness.

4. Guided Meditation:

- Listen to a guided meditation recording or app that leads you through relaxation exercises and visualizations.

- These can be particularly helpful for those new to meditation or for individuals looking for specific relaxation goals.

5. Progressive Muscle Relaxation:

- Sit or lie down and focus on a specific muscle group.

- Tense that muscle group for a few seconds, then release and let go completely.

- Move through your body, working on different muscle groups.

- This practice helps release physical tension and promotes relaxation.

CHAPTER 9

Stretching Exercises For Common Ailments

Arthritis and Joint Pain

1. Wrist Circles:

- Sit or stand with your arms extended in front of you.

- Make gentle circular motions with your wrists, moving them in a clockwise direction for 10-15 seconds.

- Then, switch to counterclockwise circles.

2. Ankle Circles:

- Sit or stand and lift one foot slightly off the ground.

- Make slow circular motions with your ankle, rotating it clockwise for 10-15 seconds.

- Reverse the direction and rotate counterclockwise.

3. Knee Lifts:

- Stand with your feet hip-width apart.

- Lift one knee towards your chest as high as comfortably possible.

- Lower it and repeat with the other knee.

- Perform 10-15 repetitions on each leg.

4. Shoulder Rolls:

- Stand or sit with your arms relaxed at your sides.

- Roll your shoulders forward in a circular motion, then reverse and roll them backward.

- Perform 10-15 repetitions in each direction.

5. Elbow Flexion and Extension:

- Sit with your arms at your sides and your palms facing forward.

- Slowly bend and straighten your elbows, keeping your palms forward.

- Perform 10-15 repetitions to improve elbow mobility.

Back Pain Relief

1. Cat-Cow Stretch:

- Start on your hands and knees.

- Inhale and arch your back (Cow pose), lifting your head and tailbone.

- Exhale and round your back (Cat pose) while tucking your chin.

- Repeat this flow for 5-10 cycles.

2. Child's Pose:

- Kneel on the floor and sit back on your heels.

- Extend your arms forward and rest your forehead on the ground.

- Hold the stretch for 15-30 seconds to release tension in your back.

3. Seated Forward Bend:

- Sit with your legs extended straight in front of you.

- Reach forward toward your toes, keeping your back straight.

- Hold the stretch for 15-30 seconds, feeling the release in your lower back.

4. Knee-to-Chest Stretch:

- Lie on your back and hug one knee to your chest.

- Hold for 15-30 seconds and switch to the other knee.

- This stretch relieves lower back tension.

5. Standing Side Stretch:

- Stand with your feet shoulder-width apart.

- Reach one arm overhead and gently bend to the side.

- Hold for 15-30 seconds on each side to stretch your side and lower back.

Stretching for Osteoporosis

1. Weight-Bearing Leg Exercises:

- Walk briskly for 30 minutes a day or engage in low-impact aerobic exercises like dancing or stair climbing to strengthen leg bones.

2. Weighted Arm Raises:

- Hold light dumbbells or water bottles in your hands.

- Stand with your arms at your sides and raise them to shoulder level.

- Lower them and repeat for 10-15 repetitions to strengthen arm bones.

3. Standing on One Leg:

- Stand near a support for balance.

- Lift one leg and balance on the other for 15-30 seconds.

- Switch legs and repeat to improve balance and strengthen leg bones.

4. Seated Leg Raises:

- Sit in a chair with your feet flat on the ground.

- Lift one leg straight in front of you and hold for a few seconds.

- Lower it and repeat with the other leg.

- Perform 10-15 repetitions on each leg.

CHAPTER 10

Stretching in Daily Life

Incorporating Stretching into Your Routine

Incorporating stretching into your daily routine is a simple yet powerful way to enhance your overall well-being. Stretching can be done at any time, and it offers numerous benefits, from reducing muscle tension to improving flexibility and posture. Here's how to seamlessly include stretching in your daily life:

1. Morning Wake-Up Stretch:

- Start your day with a few gentle stretches in bed. Reach your arms overhead and point your toes for a full-body wake-up.

2. Desk Stretch Breaks:

- Take short stretching breaks during your workday. Stand up, roll your shoulders, and stretch your arms to prevent stiffness.

3. Pre-Exercise Warm-Up:

- Incorporate dynamic stretches as a warm-up before exercise. Leg swings, arm circles, and body twists prepare your muscles for physical activity.

4. Stretch While Watching TV:

- Use TV time to perform seated or floor stretches. Reach for your toes or stretch your legs during commercials.

5. Evening Relaxation Stretch:

- Wind down in the evening with relaxation stretches. Gentle yoga or deep breathing stretches can help promote a restful night's sleep.

Stretching for Improved Sleep:

1. Child's Pose:

- Kneel on the floor and sit back on your heels.

- Extend your arms forward and rest your forehead on the ground.

- Hold for 15-30 seconds to release tension.

2. Legs Up the Wall:

- Lie on your back with your legs resting against a wall or headboard.

- Relax in this position for 5-10 minutes to reduce leg and lower back tension.

3. Supine Spinal Twist:

- Lie on your back with your arms out to the sides.

- Bend one knee and gently twist it across your body to the opposite side.

- Hold for 15-30 seconds on each side to relax your lower back and spine.

4. Seated Forward Bend:

   - Sit with your legs extended in front of you.

   - Reach forward toward your toes, keeping your back straight.

   - Hold for 15-30 seconds to relieve lower back tension.

5. Deep Breathing Stretch:

   - Sit comfortably with your eyes closed.

   - Take deep breaths and reach your arms overhead, then exhale as you bring them down.

   - Focus on your breath and stretch for 5-10 minutes to calm your mind and promote relaxation.

Incorporating stretching into your daily life, especially during key moments like morning and bedtime, can contribute to better sleep quality and overall physical and mental well-being. Experiment with different stretches to find what works best for you, and enjoy the benefits of a more flexible and relaxed body.

CONCLUSION

In the journey of life, our bodies are remarkable vessels that carry us through every experience, year after year. For seniors over 60, embracing the power of stretching exercises is more than just a practice; it's an investment in the gift of aging gracefully and healthfully.

The benefits of regular stretching exercises for seniors are numerous and invaluable. Through these exercises, you reclaim and maintain your flexibility, enabling you to move freely and without discomfort. You release the tension that accumulates over time, finding relief in the simplicity of a stretch. With improved posture, you stand tall and confident, ready to face each day with vigor.

Stretching goes beyond the physical; it offers a path to relaxation and mindfulness. As you breathe deeply and embrace the present moment, the stress of the world fades away, replaced by a sense of calm and balance. You can revel in restful nights and wake up each day with a sense of rejuvenation.

As we age, our health becomes even more precious, and regular stretching plays a pivotal role. It enhances circulation, nurtures balance, and promotes a profound connection between your body and mind.

So, to all seniors over 60, remember that you possess the power to embrace the joys of aging and cherish every moment. With each stretch, you reaffirm your commitment to a life of health, vitality, and well-being. It's never too late to begin this journey, and the benefits of regular stretching are yours to unlock.

In the graceful dance of life, stretching becomes a beautiful movement, an elegant pose in the story of your senior years. May it be a chapter filled with flexibility, vitality, and a profound sense of well-being.

FITNESS

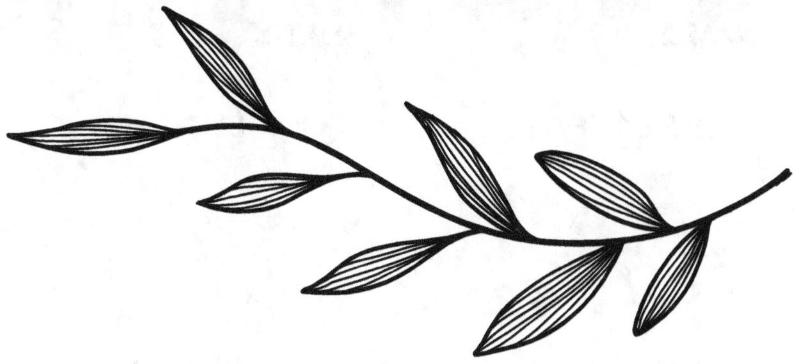

PLANNER

Fitness Planner

NAME: DATE:

BREAKFAST

LUNCH

DINNER

SNACK

EXERCISE	SET	REP	NOTES

Fitness Planner

NAME: **DATE:**

BREAKFAST

LUNCH

DINNER

SNACK

EXERCISE	SET	REP	NOTES

Fitness Planner

NAME: **DATE:**

BREAKFAST

LUNCH

DINNER

SNACK

EXERCISE	SET	REP	NOTES

Fitness Planner

NAME: **DATE:**

BREAKFAST

LUNCH

DINNER

SNACK

EXERCISE

SET   REP   NOTES

Fitness Planner

NAME: **DATE:**

BREAKFAST   ### LUNCH

DINNER   ### SNACK

EXERCISE	SET	REP	NOTES

Fitness Planner

NAME: **DATE:**

BREAKFAST

LUNCH

DINNER

SNACK

EXERCISE

SET   REP   NOTES

Fitness Planner

NAME:

DATE:

BREAKFAST

LUNCH

DINNER

SNACK

EXERCISE

EXERCISE	SET	REP	NOTES

Fitness Planner

NAME:

DATE:

BREAKFAST

LUNCH

DINNER

SNACK

EXERCISE	SET	REP	NOTES

Fitness Planner

NAME: **DATE:**

BREAKFAST   LUNCH

DINNER   SNACK

EXERCISE   SET   REP   NOTES

Fitness Planner

NAME:

DATE:

BREAKFAST

LUNCH

DINNER

SNACK

EXERCISE

SET	REP	NOTES